COD
LIVER OIL

The Essential Oil of the Ocean

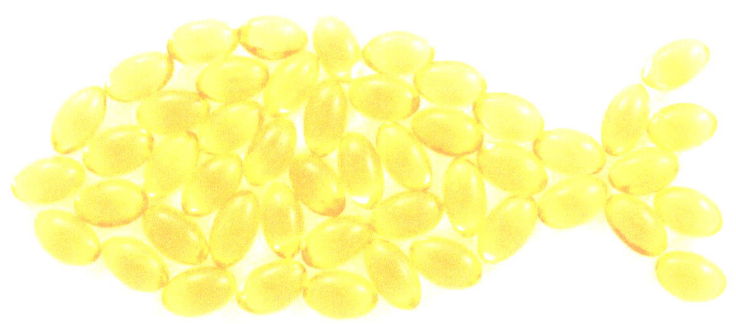

Jessica Simmons

Cod Liver Oil: The Essential Oil Of The Ocean

By Jessica Simmons

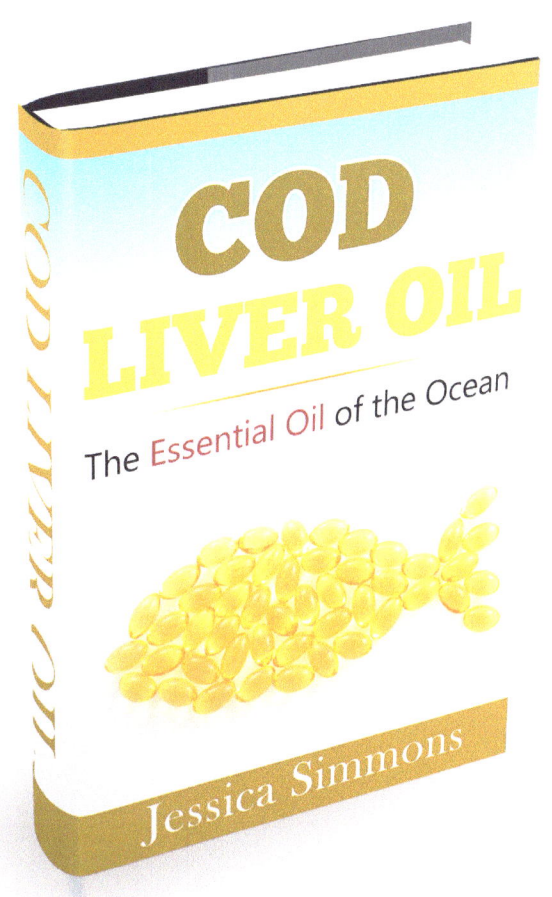

Disclaimer

Table of Contents

Introduction

I want to thank you and congratulate you for downloading the book, "Cod Liver Oil: The Essential Oil Of The Ocean."

This book contains proven steps and strategies on how to learn about the benefits of cod liver oil and the numerous benefits that it has proven to have for people. With this book, you can learn about the real reasons why cod liver oil can become such a beneficial part of your life and the specific steps and methods you can take to increase your health with it.

Cod liver oil is considered all around the world to be extremely beneficial to human health, and has been considered that way for millennia. It has long been harvested from codfish and appreciated as a remedy for low risk to serious ailments.

Cod liver oil is taken out from codfish, the meat of which is prized around the world as it contains only roughly one percent of fat. Cod liver oil is, well, the oil from the liver of a cod (hence the name, of course). Cod liver oil was instantly recognized as a beneficial source of human health and has continued to thrive that way today, and they have been made even healthier by the purification of them that has removed any harmful substances. As a result, cod liver oil is even more beneficial today than it ever was before.

As you'll discover, one reason why cod liver oil is so healthy to consume is because it is extremely high in vitamins and Omega-3 acids. In addition, cod liver oil contains much less saturated fat than other fish oils, easily making it the healthiest natural fish oil. This book will teach you all the reasons why these specific vitamins and acids are healthy to consume, and even how they can be immensely beneficial to dry skin as well.

Wait a minute; cod liver oil is a treatment for dry skin? That's right, but treating dry skin is only one of the many things that cod liver oil can remedy or alleviate the pain for. Cod liver oil can also treat and/or cure arthritis, swollen joints, heart disease, brain disease, and inflammation, diabetes, and cancer sufferers. However, there is no evidence yet that proves cod liver oil to be a cure or a true treatment for these diseases, but they may help to alleviate the pain for them. You should always speak with your doctor first before using cod liver oil, especially if you are afflicted with any of the above ailments and diseases.

However, this book will dive into specifically how and why cod liver oil has been found to alleviate the pain for such ailments, and therefore why it might be a good choice for you. For example, cod liver oil can potentially limit the chance of further developing diabetes as a result of vitamins, even though it is not a full blown cure or treatment.

Of course, with all the benefits of cod liver oil, there are also some common side effects that this book will explore as well. This will serve to give you a much better rounded view of cod liver oil instead of just a one sided viewpoint focusing only on the benefits. As you will find out, some common side effects of cod liver oils include the smell and fishy after taste of it that can give you bad breath and scent, or perhaps even cause an upset stomach and potential vomiting.

Of course, are there methods and strategies to prevent these side effects from happening? Absolutely; even if cod liver oils were a cure for cancer, many might still reconsider taking if it would give them the above symptoms and side effects, right? This book will teach you what the side effects of cod liver oils are and the different ways you can combat them.

Lastly, this book will teach you the many different ways to take cod liver oils and how to incorporate into your daily diet. If you previously thought that you had to simply take literal cod liver oil, you'd be surprised at all the different methods and ways out there to take it and use it in your daily life.

It is absolutely critical to weight the benefits of anything against the side effects. This book is written to give you a well-rounded view of cod liver oils and as much information about them as possible. Then, it will be up to you to decide whether cod liver oils are the best choice for you and whether the innumerable, proven benefits of them will outweigh the side effects (and remember that you can fight those side effects!) as well. In due course, when you finish reading this book you will have a much deeper and vaster knowledge of cod liver oils than you ever had before.

Thanks again for downloading this book, I hope you enjoy it!

Chapter 1: Where Cod Liver Oil Comes From

First of all, it's important to understand what cod liver oil is, the origins of it and where it comes from, its general history, and to get a general overview of cod liver oil and why it's been prized for entire millennia.

Cod liver oil is a nutritional supplement that comes from codfish. It is a type of fish oil, and as a result is very high in omega-3 fatty acids, and also holds high levels of Vitamin A and Vitamin D. It is specifically because of the Vitamin A and D that cod liver oil has been so prized for centuries, and the knowledge of the benefits of omega-3 fatty acids have recently come into light. Cod liver oil resembles pale yellow oil that is r\\received from the liver of the Atlantic cod. As mentioned, cod liver oil has been known about and appreciated for its health benefits for centuries. However, it first came into wide use in the 18th through the 20th centuries. It came into widespread use during this time in order to combat rickets (defective bone growth as the result of a lack of vitamin D). By the 20th Century, milk greatly increased in popularity due to the high levels of Vitamin D contained within it. This greatly helped the problem of rickets and lead to a gradual decrease of it as a decrease. Because of the usefulness of milk in combating the disease, people and doctors saw little to no need for cod liver oils anymore. However, other benefits of cod liver oils were discovered as well, such as helping heart and cardiovascular disease and arthritis, and as a result cod liver oil supplements were kept on the shelves. Later, cod liver oil was found to have a positive effect on pregnancies and for small children as well, who can benefit greatly from just a small dose each day.

Cod liver oil has been manufactured nearly as long as the benefits of it have been known. It was first manufactured through using a barrel and filing it with fresh cod livers and water. The resulting mix would form into oil after months, or in some cases even years, of mixing together. This proved to be an effective but also time consuming way to manufacture cod liver oil. Today, cod liver oil is manufactured simply by cooking the actual cod while simultaneously manufacturing fishmeal. This has proven to be a just as effective and much more time efficient method of manufacturing cod liver oils. Cod liver oil supplements are most often produced in Scandinavian countries, Iceland and Japan.

Today, cod liver oil is most often used to ease the pain and stiffness with inflammation and arthritis, to treat wounded parts of the body like skin and teeth, and to help cardiovascular and heart disease. Cod liver oil is a type of fish oil, only the benefits of cod liver oil are much greater than normal fish oils due to the very high levels of Vitamin A and Vitamin D. Just a single tablespoon of cod liver oil each day can contain enough cod liver oil to make a person healthier.

How can cod liver oil lead benefits to pregnancy? The truth is that cod liver oil is associated with a much lower risk of diabetes. The same effect can help mothers in getting enough necessary vitamins and supplements, and can also improve breast milk by increasing the level of fatty acids and Vitamin A, which reduces the risk of infections. In addition, numerous scientific studies have shown that pregnant women do benefit immensely in health reasons when it comes to cod liver oil, especially in comparison to the women who did not take the cod liver oil supplements.

Cod liver oil also contains high levels of eicosapentaenoic acid and docasahexaenoic acid, known as EPA and DHA acid respectively. These fatty acids are made in the body as a result of omega-3 acids. EPA is especially important for the body as it results in tissue hormones that are localized. DHA is also important as both the brain and the nervous system cannot function properly without it. People who are unable to produce EPA and DHA on their own as a result of nutrient deficiencies, impaired pancreatic function, consuming high amounts of polyunsaturated oils, or have diabetes may especially need a cod liver oil supplement as it is an excellent source of both.

After you purchased cod liver oil, and assuming you buy it in a bottle (as most people buy it), you should keep it safely stored in a cool, dry place. You should also be fully aware of how much of it you or your children should take, and later in this book, you will learn about the different ways that you can use cod liver oil, and how you can prepare it to make it taste better instead of simply taking it just as it is and unprepared. It's also a good idea that you keep any cod liver oil supplements that you have out of the reach of children and in a safe place.

As you'll find out in more details later, you can prepare cod liver oil in water, high vitamin butter oil, or even just regular butter. Believe it or not, but even if you mix cod liver oil with other substances, it is usually just as effective and beneficial. While your diet should always include good sources of other vitamins and minerals, making cod liver oil an important part of your diet will greatly increase your health. If you aren't convinced of the benefits, or of the arguable necessity, to take cod liver oil supplements yet, then keep on reading as we will continue to explore in much greater detail more specific benefits of it and how it can increase your health.

Now granted, there are adverse side effects that have been discovered about cod liver oil supplements over the years as well. We'll go much deeper into these side effects in a later chapter, but in this chapter we'll introduce just a few of the side effects that have come to be known about cod liver oils over time.

It's important to remember that Vitamin A gathers in the liver, and when it accumulates to increasingly high levels it can cause a little damage to the body, birth defects, an increased risk of prostate cancer in men, or a gradual increase in the overall weight of a person. Of course cod liver oil, being high in Vitamin A, can be one of the sources of accumulating large amounts of Vitamin A in the liver. This will be further explored in a later chapter, but it was one of the first side effects to be noticed about cod liver oil even as the incredible benefits of it were also becoming known.

Chapter 2: Vitamins and Minerals in Cod Liver Oil

As we have mentioned, cod liver oil is an excellent dietary supplement that will easily keep up your Vitamin A and D, and your Omega-3 Acid levels. However, many new sets of benefits have been discovered for these vitamins and acids. In addition, many new benefits about cod liver oil are being found on nearly a month to month, or even a week-to-week, basis and we are learning new things about them each day.

Generally speaking, cod liver oil is well known and well reputable for their high levels of Vitamins A and D and Omega-3 fatty acids, all of which are beneficial to the human body and are absolutely essential for anyone who otherwise hasn't had as much intake or exposure to such vitamins and acids. In all regards, people who hold cod liver oil in high regard for these reasons rightfully do so. However, even many of these people don't know why Vitamin A, Vitamin D, and Omega-3 fatty acids are so beneficial.

In addition, as we have introduced in the previous chapter, cod liver oil is also exceptionally rich in EPA and DHA acids. The human body is able to make these acids as a result from the omega-3 acids. EPA ultimately results in localized, tissue hormones because it is a critical link in a chain of fatty acids. DHA is important, as it is critical to the proper function of the brain and the nervous system. If a person is not getting enough EPA or DHA in their system one way or the other, then one reason why they should greatly consider taking cod liver oil supplements is because they are extremely rich in them.

This chapter will break down why Vitamin A and D, Omega-3 fatty acids, EPA and DHA acids are so important to the human body. Hopefully, any questions that you might have had about these vitamins and acids will be answered and further clarification about them be gotten across.

Overall, the reasons for why Vitamins A and D is beneficiary to human health vary by whatever site you visit, video you watch, doctor you talk to, or book you read. As a result, there is no real level of consistency that one can see as a result of this.

Overall, and unfortunately, the arguments for why Vitamin A is either good or bad have been greatly exaggerated in some cases for either side. Forms of synthetic Vitamin A exist in nearly any supplement, and as you can imagine, some of these supplements are better than others, and some can even be toxic! However, fat soluble Vitamin A that are found in foods are much safer and considerably less toxic than in some of the poor quality supplements…except it goes far beyond that! Vitamin A found in these foods is extremely beneficial to your body, as Vitamin A is so critical to good human health. It is very rare that toxicity would be produced by these natural Vitamin A substances, especially if it came from the cod liver oil and supplements related to cod liver oil. This is largely because the Vitamin D that is found in cod liver oil protects against the toxicity that can be found in Vitamin A. As a result, you will be able to consume a much higher amount of Vitamin A when you consume cod liver oil. Often times anyway, it's a good idea to eat a fair amount of Vitamin D when you are eating Vitamin A, and vice versa. Some foods that are rich in Vitamin D include bacon, eggs, and fish.

The incredible fact is that almost ten percent of all your genes are influenced by Vitamin D. This is why Vitamin D is so influential on your health and why it is so critical that you have high enough levels of it. Having enough Vitamin D has been found to help people from stopping the onset of a cold to preventing the flu to greatly lowering the risk of developing cancer. So as you can see, it's definitely important that you have enough of it in you, and one of the best sources of Vitamin D is from cod liver oils. Vitamin A has also been found to have a nearly equal effect on your genes, and often work together with Vitamin D. So for example, as you intake Vitamin D, it's important that you also try to intake roughly the same levels of Vitamin A. This only further reinforces why cod liver oil is so important for you, as you get roughly the same amounts of both vitamins when you consume it. Vitamin A will not be able to properly function without Vitamin D, and vice versa.

Now of course, some manufacturers of cod liver oil may add or take away certain levels of Vitamin A and Vitamin D. When you buy cod liver oil, or supplements of it, you'll want to do your best to make sure that there are enough of both vitamins within it.

It cannot be enunciated enough about how critical Vitamin A and Vitamin D are for your body's health. They directly influence your DNA via Vitamin D receptors, and as a result play a key role in preventing diseases from spreading to your body. One of the high points about Vitamin A and D is that it allows you to take control of your own health in order to largely lower the risk of developing a disease or sickness. As long as you can take the right amounts of both vitamins, you are bound to stay much healthier than the people around you. You can also spread this information to the people around you in your family, your friends, work place, and in your local neighborhood and community. For the first time in your life, you may be able to take as much control as you can over your body's health. Cod liver oil is a great source for both vitamins, and as has been stated numerous times in this book thus far, it has been proven to work.

The obvious question next is how much Vitamin A and D is necessary to consume each day. Generally speaking, 1 teaspoon for children up to the age of 12, 2 teaspoons for ages 13 to adults, and 2-3 teaspoons for pregnant women. These are generally the recommended amounts of dosage for the respective age groups. More recent research, however, has generally shown to suggest a greater necessary intake the amount of Vitamin D in order to reach the full health potential that Vitamin D can give you. If you take a lower amount of Vitamin D each day, especially during the winter, you can exhaust the stores of Vitamin D in your body extremely quickly. Maintaining optimum levels of Vitamin D in your body is crucial to reach the maximum healthy levels that Vitamin D can get you to. Therefore, it might be a good idea to intake 3-4 teaspoons worth of Vitamin D a day if you can. While 1-2 teaspoons alone should get enough Vitamin D in your body, it can just as easily burn off very quickly. If you are exposed to the sun for long periods of time, however, then consuming so much Vitamin D each day isn't as necessary as the sun alone can get you a daily dose of 5-7 teaspoons worth of Vitamin D after a period of exposure.

Therefore, if you have a job where you spend a lot of time outside in front of the sun each day, then being so concerned about Vitamin D supplements isn't so necessary. This is might even apply to Cod Liver Oils as a whole, though it's still important to get enough Vitamin A and Omega-3 acids in your body as well. It is critical to remember though, that amounts of Vitamin D in your body will increase your body's need for Vitamin A as well, and vice versa. Therefore, if you do decide you don't need Cod Liver Oil supplements based on the amount of Vitamin D you're already getting, then you can always eat other sources of Vitamin A such as eggs, butter fats, chicken and fish.

If you are not sure about how much Vitamin A and D you are getting, then you can always get your levels of each tested. This is highly recommended if you are especially unsure of your levels of either vitamin and if you are unsure if taking cod liver oil supplements will be necessary.

Chapter 3: The Benefits of Cod Liver Oil

Now that we have gone over the different, specific minerals and acids within cod liver oil, and how they work and are good for the body's health, then how is cod liver oil itself beneficial to the body? After all, all that the last chapter explained was why Vitamin A and D, and Omega-3 acids are critical for the body's health. And cod liver oil is an excellent source for those vitamins and acids, right? Correct. But aren't there other sources of Vitamin A and D and Omega-3 acids? Absolutely there are. So why then, is Cod Liver Oil in particular, so beneficial to the body and human health? What makes it stand apart from the other sources of these vitamins and acids that are so beneficial?

First of all, when someone mentions the term 'Cod Liver Oil,' your first reaction may be "gross!" That's a perfectly valid reaction…and perhaps the one reason why you or someone else may seriously be considering another source of the beneficial vitamins and acids. But if history and science have shown anything, it's that cod liver oil itself is one of the best sources of these acids. This chapter will explain why.

As we discussed before, cod liver oil has been used as a source of food and as a beneficiary for human health for millennia. It has been used so all the way back since the days of the Roman Empire. The sciences of today have dissected the 'ingredients' within it that make it so beneficial (as we explored in the last chapter). But the truth remains that you will have to dig hard to find a more beneficiary source to human health that is as natural as cod liver oil. Sure, you'll find plenty of supplements recommended by your doctors that may work better. But if you want to stick with natural sources, then cod liver oil is the way to go.

Yes, the Omega-3 fatty acids produce high amounts of EPA and DHA acids, and the high levels of Vitamin A and Vitamin D together make cod liver oil such an efficient and easy source of both. Indeed, many other biological processes entirely depend on these acids and vitamins. Each water-soluble vitamin and mineral uptake requires Vitamin A, and Vitamin A cannot suffice without roughly equal levels of Vitamin D. Cod liver oil delivers BOTH, something that many other supplements are unable to do, or at least not to the extent of cod liver oil. In addition, both vitamins, and Vitamin D in particular, are especially necessary for those who live in places where there isn't as much sunlight. The single greatest sources of Vitamin D are from the sun, and if the sun isn't coming out as often anytime soon, that's when you need to turn to other sources. And again, there are very few sources, natural or synthetic, that are as effective as cod liver oil.

Simply put, cod liver oil contains extremely large amounts of Vitamin A, Vitamin D and Omega-3 fatty acids. All of these nutrients are absolutely essential and are difficult to obtain in a typical, American diet. Synthetic substances are also untrustworthy, so you have to do your research there to determine which companies are good and which ones aren't. This is often a long and confusing process, and besides, you may want to use natural sources instead. If you do, then besides sunlight, there is no greater natural source of these acids and vitamins than cod liver oils. Why? Because cod liver oil contains more Vitamin A and D than any other food. Even though we typically consume cod liver oil in smaller amounts, it only takes a tablespoon of cod liver oil to get the necessary Vitamin A, Vitamin D and Omega-3 fatty acids into our bodies.

Throughout history and even through scientific, medical test, there are very few diseases that react poorly with cod liver oil. This applies to diseases and illnesses ranging from the common cold to the flu to heart disease to even cancer. Of course, this is attributed to the vitamins and acids contained within cod liver oil. But you never know, as we continue to discover new things with science every day, we could possibly find out even more reasons behind the beauty of cod liver oil. Almost every disease and illness has reacted well with cod liver oil.

Okay, so we get the point. Cod liver oil is extremely beneficiary to human health. Both history and medical science of the present day have shown that there are no other foods or supplements that contain as high levels of Vitamin A and Vitamin D, and Omega-3 acids as cod liver oil, and there are very few illnesses or diseases that don't react well with cod liver oil. Does that mean that everyone should take cod liver oil?

Yes! This is another huge benefit to cod liver oil, as anyone can take it. It is highly effective in both adults and children alike. As long as you start with the necessary dosages of a ½ teaspoon of cod liver oil for children, then 1 teaspoon for teenagers to adults, and roughly 2 teaspoons (or more) for pregnant women, then cod liver oil will work for nearly anyone.

There are also many manufacturers that you can buy cod liver oil from. When you do buy from a manufacturer, it's important that you do your research and buy from a manufacturer that utilizes a traditional method of fermenting oil, instead of through high temperature processing. As a result, more of the nutrients, vitamins and acids are preserved in the cod liver oil this way. Most importantly, the ratio of Vitamin A to Vitamin D is preserved through this method as well.

You also have to watch out for brands of cod liver oil that have been highly processed as a result of the manufacturing. The cod liver oil that has gone through this process will not be as effective due to losing its critical and acid content. Some manufacturers will even add synthetic vitamins back in to the cod liver oil in order to make up for the vitamins and acids that were lost, but not even these synthetic vitamins are as effective as the natural ones.

Overall, you will want to buy from a manufacturer that uses an old-fashioned fermentation method in the manufacturing of the cod liver oil, as this is the only way you can make sure that the important vitamins and acids are preserved and that the ratio of Vitamin A to D is preserved. This will require some extra research, so you may want to consult with your doctor and talk to friends and family members who have cod liver oil in the past to get their preferences. From there, you can narrow your list of potential brands to buy and wrap up your research by reading the facts about the cod liver oil brand to find out if it uses the traditional fermentation method. If so, then it's a good bet that the manufacturer has the correct, ratio of Vitamin A to Vitamin D.

So let's say that after your research, you finally find a manufacturer that makes cod liver oil using the traditional fermentation method, but now you can't afford it. It is absolutely critical that you get the necessary vitamins and acids in you, and since cod liver oil is by far one of the best sources for that, it's important that you at least try to get the best cod liver oil that you can. You can always turn to a synthetic cod liver oil if you can't afford the good, natural oils, but the synthetic cod liver oils simply aren't near as effective as the natural.

Fortunately though, the good, natural cod liver oil usually isn't as expensive as it may sound. Keep in mind too, that you only need to take smaller doses each day, so buying a bottle for $50 should last you a long time. You can also attempt to buy the best manufacturer for the money if the best of the best is simply more money than you are able to spend.

The benefits of cod liver oil truly is incredible, and most of the times even the best bottles shouldn't be too expensive anyway. There simply is no other source that will get you high enough levels and the right balance of Vitamin A and Vitamin D into your body, let alone the Omega-3 acids as well. As there are a very limited number of illnesses and diseases that cannot be helped by cod liver oil, it is an excellent natural source for anyone to take…and it literally works for anyone.

The last benefit of cod liver oil is that it can help to relieve dry skin. Dry skin can cause excessive itchiness and is very bothersome to the people who have it. One of the best ways to fight cod liver oil is to apply a cream that contains cod liver oil to the dry skinned area. Think of this as the same way of using the lotions and moisturizers that you are already using. After getting out of the shower, when your skin is still moist, adding a cod liver oil cream to the dry skinned area is one of the best ways to stop it and to prevent it from happening again in the future.

In addition, simply taking cod liver oil itself, without mixing it with a cream or applying it to your dry skin directly, can also prevent the onset of dry skin. However, this method is not as effective as applying the cod liver oil to the dry skin directly.

Of course, however, there are potential side effects that can result from cod liver oil, and this book would simply not be a fair assessment if it were to not include the side effects as well to help give you a better rounded view of cod liver oils. This next chapter will dive just into that, and in due course you should be able to weigh the positives against the negatives to help decide whether cod liver oil is the right choice for you.

Chapter 4: Potential Side Effects of Cod Liver Oil

This chapter will dive into the potential side effects that can result from cod liver oil. First of all, as we have gone over, the benefits of cod liver oil truly are extraordinary. It has proven itself to be an effective resistance against diseases and illnesses alike over hundreds of years, and it is a great supplement for Vitamin A and D, and omega 3 acids. Cod liver oil will be immensely beneficial for your immune system, cancer, asthma, brain, heart and joints, and can also help against inflammation.

So now that we fully understand the benefits of cod liver oil, it's time that we discuss the side effects and negatives that are commonly associated with it. In the previous chapter, we talked about the effectiveness of the natural fermentation process and how it can help to preserve the vitamins and acids in it. This is true, but also much oil can be lost in this process, causing most manufacturers to add a chemical solvent to the oil and to heat the liver to over four hundred degrees. While the chemical solvent is intended to bind the oil, traces of the chemical still remain inside the cod liver oil even in the best cod liver oils that you could find on the market. Even in these, there are some synthetic vitamins that will have to be added to the oil, due to the process of chemical extraction and synthetic vitamins. So unfortunately, the number of 'good' cod liver oil manufacturers is slowly but gradually dwindling.

Cod liver oil contains concentrated doses of Omega-3 acids. Omega-3 fatty acids can greatly aid in fighting inflammation in the joints and leading to overall lower cholesterol levels. This can help to greatly reduce the chance of heart disease, arthritis, strokes, chronic diseases, and brain damage (all major positives), but there are still some side effects that come with cod liver oil that that go beyond the simple negatives of manufacturer errors.

Often times after consuming cod liver oil, one many have a fishy aftertaste. Cod liver oil that comes in capsules attempt to solve the problem of the fishy after taste by being in a capsule itself and containing anti-odor supplements, but the capsule can only protect against the fishy after taste in the mouth. The capsule will break down in the stomach, and even though it's a good thing that it releases the cod liver oil inside, belching and rising stomach acids will ensure leading to heartburn and a fishy taste that develops at the throat. Granted, there is a way that you can help fight this fishy aftertaste regardless of whether or not you take the cod liver oil in a capsule or not. If you take cod liver oil along with your food and do not lie down right after eating the food and taking the cod liver oil, then you can greatly reduce the chance of having the fishy aftertaste. And as a result, you'll also have better breath!

Something else to keep in mind about a fishy aftertaste resulting from cod liver oil is that it can vary by the manufacturer or brand that you buy from. It can also vary by how you take the cod liver oil, such as whether by capsule, pill or in a liquid form.

Another problem that can arise with cod liver oil is disturbances within the digestive system. This goes hand in hand with the belching and heartburn talk about in the last paragraph. Besides the belching and heartburn that will lead to a fishy aftertaste at your throat, you could also potentially feel a stomach ache, bloating and nausea leading to vomiting and diahrrea. This doesn't sound very much fun, now does it. And it's certainly a negative side effect to weight against the benefits of cod liver oil as well. But as with nearly any side effect, there are ways that you can try to prevent these digestive problems from occurring. The two best methods are to take cod liver oil in a capsule, as doing so will greatly reduce the risk of these extended digestive problems that go beyond the belching and heartburn from occurring. In addition, your body will have to get used to cod liver oil, so you must give your body some time to adjust to it. If you use these two methods, they are the best ways to protect against these bad digestive problems.

As we have discussed, cod liver oil are useful for preventing heart and cardiovascular disease. It is able to do this by thinning the blood to slow blood clotting. Unfortunately, lowering the blood clotting can also increase the risk of bleeding. The best way to fight this side effect is to consult with your doctor to see if there are any additional medications that you can take to prevent the bleeding from taking place. Your doctor may or may not advise that you take cod liver oil capsules and supplements.

While taking cod liver oil in the form of a capsule is a good idea to prevent digestive problems, it has been found that even taking it in the form of a capsule can also still have the side effect of raising blood sugar levels. Scientific studies have been conducted that show that blood sugar levels have actually increased as a result of consuming cod liver oils, and even when it was taken in the form of a capsule. As with bleeding, the best way to fight this side effect is to consult with your doctor first to see if there is any additional medication that you can take to decrease your blood sugar levels.

Another side effect that can potentially come from cod liver oil is an unfortunate result of our oceans being polluted. As the amount of trash and junk being dumped into our oceans has increased in recent decades, this means that the cod can consume hazardous materials with links to cancer before they are caught. Fortunately, cod liver oil itself can greatly help prevent the spread of cancer in the body, or even possibly prevent it entirely, but it's still important to keep in mind that the fish could have consumed hazardous materials.

Now that you know the benefits and the side effects of using cod liver oil, it's ultimately up to you to weight those benefits against the side effects and determine whether or not taking cod liver oil is the right choice for you. Something to keep in mind, however, is that the methods we have discussed to fight the side effects have been proven to work, so it's also critically important to take those methods into consideration as well.

Chapter 5: Ways to Use Cod Liver Oil

So far we have discussed with cod liver oil is, the important vitamins and acids contained within it, the benefits of using it, and the side effects that are ultimately associated with it. It's up to you to weight the benefits against the side effects (and the methods to help prevent the potential side effects from occurring). But assuming that you want to proceed and take cod liver oil, the question most likely on your mind is how to take it. Do you take cod liver oil as a pill, or a gel, or a liquid, etc.? There are numerous ways that you can take cod liver oils and also many different ways to use it as well. That's what this chapter is going to discuss.

One way you can take cod liver oil is to take it in a liquid form and add it to your favorite kind of juice. You can then gulp it down! For this way of taking it, you should find the best flavor of cod liver oil that you can, since even mixing a poor flavor with your favorite juice will be difficult to gulp down all in one sitting. And hey, not everyone like's juice. You can always mix it in with something else like a smoothie as well.

There are also blended cod liver oils that you can take as well. These blended oils are often more expensive, but they taste much better too. If you have sensitive taste buds, then blended cod liver oils are probably the best way to go. But even with blended cod liver oils, it's always a good idea to have a glass of water or your favorite snack on standby to consume immediately after the cod liver oils. It's generally healthier to eat or drink with cod liver oils anyway, and it will be easier to consume as well. Organically flavored cod liver oils go hand in hand with blended cod liver oils, with many flavors such as cinnamon, mint, or licorice.

One of the best ways to take cod liver oil is in the form of a capsule, as it is tasteless and also the healthiest way to take it to see the best results. As long as you eat a meal when you take the capsule, you shouldn't be a victim of the infamous fishy aftertaste as well. If there is one downside to taking cod liver oil as a capsule, it is that it is a generally more expensive way of taking it. However, many people are willing to spend the extra money if it means that taking a capsule is the most effective way to fully take in all the health benefits of cod liver oil, and to receive the fewest side effects as well.

You can also take cod liver oil by simply pouring it into a spoon and taking it that way. Simply hold your breath and swallow. Of course, this method does require a lot of courage, but many people do report that this method means that you can hardly take the cod liver oil anyway. Plus, you take it just as it is without mixing it in with any other substances.

You can also put the cod liver oil in a glass of water and drink it with one, big swallow as well. This is similar to the spoon method, but can lead to less of a taste while swallowing, and also means that you don't risk mixing the cod liver oil with the supplements in the juice if you would rather have gone with the juice method.

Besides, who said that you had to mix cod liver oil with water or juice? You can also always try mixing it with yogurt, raw cream, half and half, or you can even try blending it with raw honey and maple syrup as well. Other options that go hand in hand with this include blending it with salad dressing (and can actually add taste to an otherwise dull, typical salad), or with vegetables like a lemon slice or a cucumber. Just chewing vegetables immediately after taking the cod liver oil can make all the difference when it comes to taste!

Another method that we have talked about is to mix the cod liver oil with a cream and then apply it directly to dry skin. Even if you don't have any dry skin that requires cod liver oil, simply applying cod liver oil directly to healthy skin is one way to absorb the nutrients if you don't want to take it orally. The only downside to this method is that not all the nutrients, such as the vitamins and acids, would be absorbed if you otherwise chose to take it orally.

But regardless of the way that you choose to take cod liver oil, you should always try to take it with a positive attitude. If you have a poor or negative attitude when taking cod liver oil, then chances are you won't like it and it will be only more difficult for you take it in the future. Simply having positive emotions can make all the difference on your brain when you take cod liver oil, and help your body to absorb all the more beneficial nutrients of it as well.

As you can see, all that it really takes is a little bit of creativity for taking cod liver oil. Taking it due to the poor taste of it may scare some people, but the many different ways that you can take cod liver oil are not as limited as some people may try to tell you. Plus, the ways you can take it that you have learned do not disrupt the high level of vitamins and acids within cod liver oil, or the proper balance of Vitamin A and Vitamin D.

The best cod liver oils to take are the ones that are high in Vitamin A and Vitamin D. Of course, many manufactured cod liver oils completely lack these vitamins and the Omega-3 acids. When you take cod liver oils, you should conduct heavy research to find a brand that doesn't manufacture their cod liver oil to the point that they have to use vitamin supplements to replace the Vitamin A and D that has been lost in the manufacturing process. One of the best brands to buy is from Green Pasture, as the cod liver oil made by his manufacturer isn't manufactured to the point that all the important vitamins and acids are lost.

Another plus about Green Pasture cod liver oil is that it is made through the natural fermentation process. This means that the cod liver oil is as authentic as possible throughout the production process. The unheated cod liver oil that is offered in small batches is often the form of cod liver oil that maintains the healthy 'ingredients.'

Chapter 6: Common Questions about Cod Liver Oil

At this point, we have gone over nearly all the information that there is to know about cod liver oil: what it is; the specific nutrients, vitamins and acids within it; the benefits and side effects of it; and the most common and effective ways to take it. This chapter will wrap up this book and answer some common questions that exist about cod liver oil.

- How much cod liver oil should one take?
  - Generally speaking, ½ teaspoon for children, 1 – 2 teaspoons for adults, and 3 – 4 teaspoons for pregnant women.
- Is Cod Liver Oil colorless?
  - No, not entirely. Vitamin A is indeed colorless, but cod liver oil tends to be either an orange, yellow or brown color.
- Is it true that cod liver oil can make you belch? How can you prevent that?
  - It is true for some people, depending on the person. The best thing you can do is to take your cod liver oil in the form of a capsule, and to take it while you are eating a meal. Also avoid lying or sitting down immediately after you have taken it. If none of these methods work, then consult your doctor.
- Do you have to have a sufficient calcium intake before taking cod liver oil?
  - It is generally a good idea, yes. It's generally a good idea to get about 1,000 – 2,500 mg of calcium in you each day before taking cod liver oil supplements.

- If codfish oil is fish oil, then doesn't that mean that it will disrupt the balance of omega-3 and omega-6 acids as most fish oils do? After all, doctors' right does generally not recommend fish oils?

  - Cod liver oil is a fish oil, but it is also a much different type of fish oil and much more beneficial to the human body. Cod liver oil is most renowned for the high levels and having a right balance of Vitamin A and Vitamin D. However, you also get enough omega fatty acids, and especially enough of Omega-3, if you take the right amount of daily doses of cod liver oil. The balance between Omega-3 and Omega-6 fatty acids shouldn't be disrupted. As for what doctors do or do not recommend, it largely depends on the type of fish oil and the doctor, but cod liver oil is by far the most beneficial fish oil that there is to human health.

- Don't most fish diets contain high levels of mercury and other heavy metals that are harmful to human health? Wouldn't this be included in cod liver oils as well?

  • A lot of fish does contain mercury, and it is mostly stored in the protein of the fish and not in the fat, which is where cod liver oil comes from. Even if the cod liver oil you consume does have mercury levels in it, the Vitamin A in it is an excellent defense against mercury and other toxic, hard metal substances that could be contained within the fish as well. This is also a good defense against other diets you eat that may contain high levels of mercury within it.

- Will cod liver oil cause damage to bone and bone structure?

  • No, absolutely not. On the contrary, cod liver oil is actually quite beneficial to strengthening bones and joints in particular. Vitamin A and Vitamin D are both very protective of bone structure, especially if the ratio between both of the two vitamins is consistent. People with the highest levels of Vitamin A and Vitamin D in their systems are the least likely to feel pain between their joins or risk a bone fracture.

- Let's say that you are working a job where you are very much exposed to the sun all day long, and you are also taking cod liver oil supplements to get enough Vitamin A, Vitamin D and Omega-3 acids into your body…but the sun is the best source of Vitamin D. Does this mean that you could be getting too much Vitamin D into your body, and what are the effects of that?

- It is possible that you could overdose on Vitamin D, so if you really are exposed to the sun all day long, then you may want to consider cutting back on the cod liver oil supplements you are taking. Or, you could completely stop taking cod liver oils and take other supplements to get Vitamin A and Omega-3 fatty acids into your body, but it's especially important that the ratio between Vitamin A and Vitamin D in your body is consistent if you want to remain healthy. The best thing you can do here is to consult your doctor to first find out the levels of Vitamin A and Vitamin D that are in your body first, and once you get a sense of what your levels are, you can go from there. In general in this situation though, it would be a good idea to scale back on how much cod liver oil you take. If you are an adult, you should consider scaling back from your original daily dosage of 1 – 2 teaspoons to about ¾ of a teaspoon per day. You should also consider always check on your levels throughout the process to make sure that you do not overdose or under dose on anything. There are limits on the safety of cod liver oil no doubt, and that would include not overdosing on Vitamin D if you are exposed to the sun all day. More modern cod liver oils, however, have been found to be safer than older ones, as there is not as much oxidation within them. Even so, consider a ¾ teaspoon of cod liver oil per day to the maximum amount you should take if you are exposed to the sun all day. Just check up on your levels and consult your doctor throughout the process and you should be fine.

- Is cod liver oil only effective because of the high amounts of omega-3 acids that are contained within it?

- No. While omega-3 acids are contained within cod liver oil and they are highly beneficial, Vitamin A and Vitamin D also plays a huge role in the benefits of cod liver oil for human health. However, you should be aware that some commercial cod liver oils are manufactured in a non-fermented way, meaning that they can lose some of the Vitamin A and Vitamin D within it and be replaced by synthetic Vitamin A and D. In this case, the Omega-3 acids would be the real beneficiary part of the cod liver oil, but as long as you buy fermented cod liver oil, then Vitamin A and Vitamin D will play a far greater role than Omega-3 acids. Unfortunately, a lot of the cod liver oils that you can buy in the store today are not the naturally fermented ones.

- Wouldn't adding cod liver oil to your daily diet drastically increase the amount of calories you intake? If omega-3 acids are fats, and since fats contain a large amount of calories, then people taking cod liver oils each day would technically be increasing the amount of calories they intake each day, right? Does this mean that if you want to take cod liver oils for its health benefits, which you would have to change your daily diet?

  - No. Many people assume that eating fatter is unhealthy. That is true…depending the fat. Rather than simply saying that fats are unhealthy and thus must be avoided, it would be far better to break down what specific kinds of fats are healthy and which ones aren't. In fact, many people can develop illnesses and diseases as a result of a lack of nutrients that are found in fats and reduce fat intake. There are many soluble nutrients that are found in fats and hardly anywhere else in a typical diet. These include a variety of Vitamin A's, Vitamin D's, Vitamin E's, and Vitamins K. These also include plant stem cells, hormones, and enzymes. The important thing to remember when wanting to avoid illnesses and diseases is to watch on how much sugar you intake and to eat healthy fats. Healthy fats can come outside grazing chickens, livestock, and fish eggs.

- Cod liver oil is extremely rich in Vitamin A and Vitamin D. Aren't Vitamin A and Vitamin D unsafe if they are taken in large amounts?

  • It is true that large amounts of Vitamin A and D can be unsafe, and it's also critical that when you do consume Vitamin A and D, that the ratio between the two is proportional. However, it's also important to remember that your body won't be very healthy without Vitamin A and Vitamin D. Cod liver oil is one of the best sources of that in the world. As long as you take the recommended doses of cod liver oil, you won't get too much or too little of Vitamin A and D, so you have nothing to worry about there. It's also important that you take fermented cod liver oil, as this is the traditional and most effective way to produce cod liver oil and preserve Vitamin A and Vitamin D in it. More commercial methods lead to a loss of Vitamin A and D in the cod liver oil, and as a result, synthetic vitamins that will not deliver you the necessary nutrients for good health supplement them.

- Should people who have diabetes only use cod liver oil if a doctor or medical professional supervises them?

  • It's always a good idea to at least consult your doctor first. However, many people think that cod liver oil can only make people with diabetes worse. The truth is that this entirely depends on the type of cod liver oil you receive. Commercial cod liver oil is not fermented the traditional way, and as a result loses its original, natural Vitamin A and D. These vitamins are replaced by synthetic vitamins, which can cause more harm than good to people with diabetes. However, very little is actually know about this subject, so more research by scientists and medical professionals over the coming the years should yield more information about this.

Conclusion

Thank you again for downloading this book!

I hope this book was able to help you to understand what cod liver oil is; where it comes from; the benefits and side effects of it; how it can be used and common questions that many people have about cod liver oil.

This book was intended to be a general overview of the facts of cod liver oil. Hopefully you were able to now understand all you need to know about cod liver oil and decide whether it is best for you. The benefits of cod liver oil truly are exceptional and are unrivaled by any other natural sources. They have been used for millennia as a means to prevent or treat illnesses and diseases, and the findings we have made in science and the medical field in recent years has only further reinforced the fact that cod liver oil is an exceptional choice for anyone to take.

The next step is for you to decide whether or not cod liver oil is the right choice for you. You have to weigh the benefits of it against the side effects, but you must also keep in mind the tools and methods in this book to help prevent the potential side effects of it as well. You should always consult with your doctor throughout the process and always check in on your levels of Vitamin A and Vitamin D, and talk to any friends or family members who have taken or are familiar with cod liver oil to get their assessment of it.

Lastly, always remember the kind of cod liver oil that you are buying. If you don't buy the naturally fermented kind, you'll consume synthetic, unnatural Vitamin A and Vitamin D and won't reap the true benefits of cod liver oil. In that case, you might think that everything in this book was junk! That is why you must try to buy natural, fermented cod liver oil. And then, in due course, you will unlock and discover the true benefits behind cod liver oil and realize how beneficial it truly is. At that point, you can count yourself as one of the many different people throughout history and the present day who have enjoyed the benefits of what it can do for human health.

Good luck to you as you embark on your journey towards getting a more healthy body. You can and will succeed as long as you successfully apply the steps, tips and tools that this book has taught you. And who knows, maybe you'll be the one telling your friends and family members all about what cod liver oil can do for them!

Finally, if you enjoyed this book, please take the time to share your thoughts and post a review on Amazon. It'd be greatly appreciated!